Handy Note on Leukemia

Coping Strategies and Treatment Insights; Knowledge at Your Fingertips.

Emily R. Williams

Dedication

This book is dedicated to God Almighty for the success of this work. It is also dedicated to all Leukaemia patients out there.

There is hope! There is a bright future ahead!

Table of Content

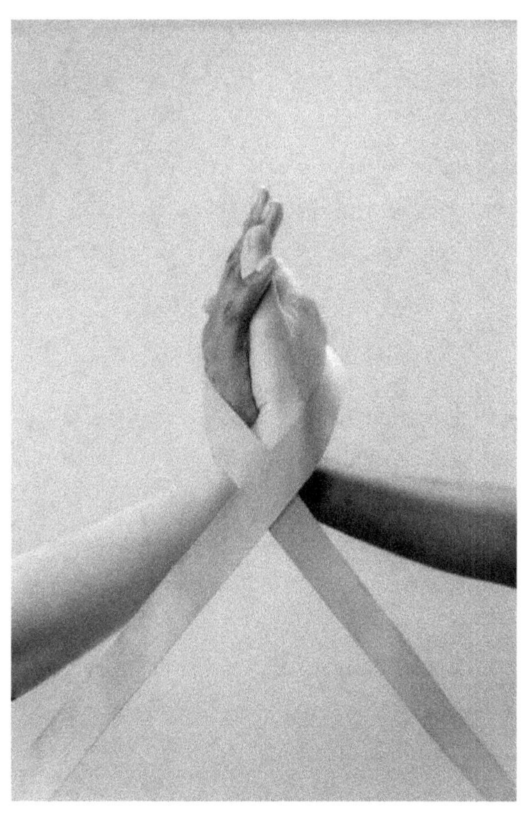

Introduction

In the past, bright banners with the words "Unite for a Cure - Together We Rise!" decorated the walls of a small town named Hopeville. Young and old residents of the town congregated in the town center to hear the most recent updates from the Hopeville Research Center, where the most brilliant brains toiled nonstop to find a treatment for leukemia.

Emily, a lively young girl with golden curls, dazzling eyes, and a contagious laugh that made everyone around her smile, lived at the center of this thriving village. Emily had been identified as having leukemia, thus a shadow loomed beneath her radiant grin. The news sent shockwaves through the entire community since Emily served as Hopeville's beating heart, and the idea of her suffering was intolerable.

The residents of Hopeville, though, were not easily overcome. They came together, resolved to stand by Emily and discover a treatment that would revive her vivacious energy. The town's scientists, physicians, and researchers set out to solve the riddles of leukemia, motivated by this shared objective. Their lab transformed into a haven of hope as the days grew into months, and their commitment stoked the flames of research.

Among the microscopes and test tubes, a young researcher named Alex became engrossed in an original concept. What if they could harness the immune system's power to fight leukemia? This idea motivated Alex to put forth many hours of research into the nuances of immunotherapy. He was certain that it had the key to learning the mysteries of the ailment.

To promote leukemia research, the community in Hopeville's center planned a number of fundraisers and activities. Grandma Millie's lemon cake was a popular item at a charity bake-off where they also conducted music festivals and art auctions. Motivated by the conviction that, when unified, they could overcome anything, the entire community came together as one.

One pleasant summer evening, Emily sat on her porch and looked up at the starry sky as the sun sunk below the horizon. Hope that a cure might be discovered soon made her heart flutter. Her closest friend, Tim, reassured her, "You're going to beat this, Emily," by gently squeezing her hand. Emily nodded as she felt the depth of their connection saturate her.

At the Hopeville Research Center, Alex's experiment had produced a significant advance. He figured out how to direct T-cells, the immune system's soldiers, to specifically target leukemia cells. His coworkers gave him a standing ovation for this amazing discovery, but he knew the real joy would come when it helped Emily and others in a similar situation.

As news of Alex's success went across the community, Hopeville was a hive of activity. The populace understood that something unusual was about to happen. The research facility was humming with activity as plans were being made for the revolutionary clinical experiment that would alter people's lives forever.

Emily signed up for the clinical trial with a renewed sense of hope, eager to take part in the leukemia treatment revolution. The entire community came together to support their heroic heroine, standing as one force behind her.

The sun rose on the day of the trial at a significant moment. As Emily entered the research facility with her eyes gleaming with resolve, the neighborhood had gathered there and was waving banners of support. She was escorted into the chamber where her T-cells would be re-engineered by Alex, who was both excited and anxious.

As the trial therapy started, the symphony of optimism reached its peak. Emily signed up for the clinical trial with a renewed sense of hope, eager to take part in the leukemia treatment revolution. The entire community came together to support their heroic heroine, standing as one force behind her.

Emily viewed the lively town of Hopeville from the top of the hill one sunny morning. "Hope Lives Here" has taken the place of the previous banner that read, "Unite for a Cure – Together We Rise!" She was aware that her encounter had sparked an iota of hope that would reverberate for generations to come. The battle against leukemia has come to an end, or better yet, a new chapter has begun.

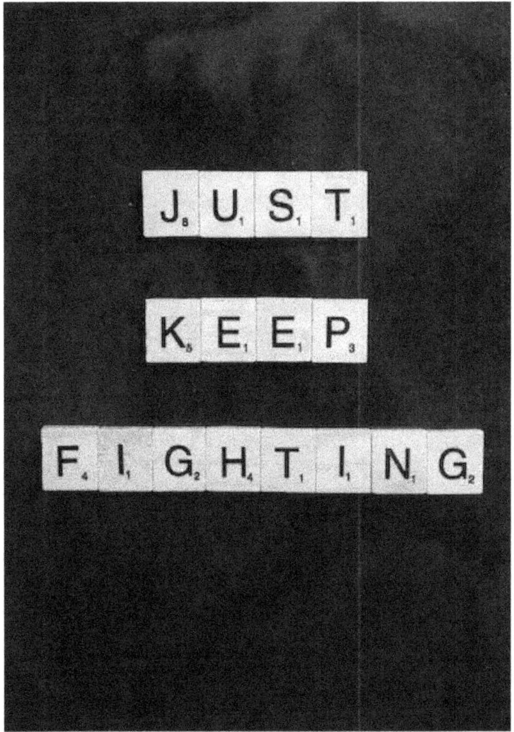

As a result, the tale of Hopeville came to represent bravery, love, and the unbreakable spirit of mankind. A reminder that even the worst of circumstances could be overcome by hope and unity.

Chapter 1

Understanding Leukemia

→ Definition

White blood cell production is abnormally increased in leukemia, a blood and bone marrow malignancy. Normally, white blood cells play a major role in the body's defense against illnesses and infections. However, these cells deteriorate and stop working in leukemia. The bone marrow becomes overworked as a result of their quick growth and is unable to create healthy blood cells like platelets and red blood cells.

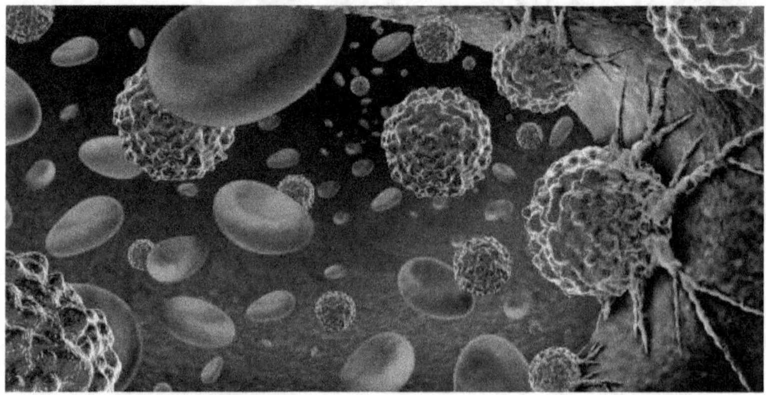

→ General Overview

There are two fundamental types of leukemia that can be identified depending on how quickly the disease progresses:

Acute leukemia: This type of the illness progresses swiftly and results in a quick development of immature, abnormal white blood cells (blasts) in the bone marrow and blood. Acute leukemia requires immediate and aggressive treatment.

Chronic Leukemia: White blood cells that are abnormally formed and increase more slowly in chronic leukemia. Before the disease gets worse, it could take months or even years. In certain cases, waiting it out is a viable option for treating persistent leukemia

It can also be classified based on the type of white blood cell affected by leukemia:

A type of white blood cell called acute lymphocytic leukemia (ALL) affects lymphocytes, which are involved in the immune system.

Acute myeloid leukemia (AML) affects myeloid cells, which are the precursors of red blood cells, platelets, and particular types of white blood cells.

Elderly people are more likely to develop Chronic Lymphocytic Leukaemia (CLL), which affects mature lymphocytes.

A characteristic of chronic myeloid leukemia (CML), which affects mature myeloid cells, is the Philadelphia chromosome.

Leukaemia can affect anyone at any age, however some kinds are more common in certain age groups.

Chapter 2

An explanation of its prevalence and negative consequences on health

Prevalence

Leukaemia is a kind of cancer that is quite common, accounting for around 3% of all cancer cases globally. All ages are impacted, but adults are more likely than kids to experience it. Leukaemia might be more common in some places than others, depending on the type and locale. Acute leukemias, such as acute myeloid leukemia (AML) and acute lymphocytic leukemia (ALL), are often more common in children and young adults. However, chronic myeloid leukemia (CML) and chronic lymphocytic leukemia (CLL) diagnoses are more common in older patients.

Leukaemia has a major negative impact on a person's health and wellbeing in a variety of ways. These include:

Physical Health: Because leukemia prevents the bone marrow from producing blood cells normally, anemia, a drop in platelets (which increases the risk of bleeding), and an accumulation of aberrant white blood cells are all side effects. Weakness, recurring infections, easily bleeding and bruising, and tiredness are possible signs and symptoms of this.

Emotional and Psychological Impact: Receiving a leukemia diagnosis can be emotionally trying for the sufferer as well as their loved ones. The unpredictable nature of the condition, the tight treatment regimens, and the fear of passing away can all lead to stress, anxiety, and despair.

Nausea, vomiting, hair loss, tiredness, and an increased susceptibility to infections are examples of treatment adverse effects. Leukemia treatments that are frequently used include chemotherapy and radiation therapy. These side effects may have a negative influence on the patient's quality of life during and after therapy.

<u>Financial Burden</u>: Leukaemia treatment can be expensive, which puts a heavy financial burden on patients and their families. High medical costs that are difficult to manage may emerge from the need for ongoing treatment and supportive care.

<u>Effect on Daily Life</u>: Leukaemia and its treatment may make it more difficult for a person to engage in regular activities including job, study, and recreation. Patients may need to take time off from work or school for therapy and recovery. Relapse is always a possibility, which can be emotionally challenging for patients and their families even if some varieties of leukemia can be properly treated.

Despite these challenges, advances in leukemia research and treatment throughout the years have led to better outcomes for many patients. Early detection and rapid treatment remain crucial for managing the illness and improving long-term survival chances.

Leukemia sufferers must have a strong support system that includes medical professionals, family, and friends in order to cope with the physical and emotional challenges of the disease. Regular monitoring and follow-up care are essential to effectively manage the condition and provide individuals with leukemia with the highest quality of life possible.

Chapter 3

Acute Leukemia

➢ **Acute Lymphoblastic Leukemia (ALL)**

Acute lymphoblastic leukemia (ALL), which is also called acute lymphocytic leukemia, is a type of cancer that affects the white blood cells called lymphocytes. It is the most frequent kind of leukemia in children, although being less common in adults. ALL is characterized by the rapid maturation of immature lymphocytes, or lymphoblasts, in the bone marrow and the subsequent accumulation of these cells in the blood and other organs.

Causes and chance Factors: Although there is no known cause for ALL, a number of factors have been associated with a higher chance of developing this type of leukemia, including:

Genetic Predisposition: In certain situations, chromosomal abnormalities or genetic mutations may aid in the development of ALL.

Exposure to Ionizing Radiation or Specific Carcinogenic Chemicals: High levels of exposure to ionizing radiation or particular carcinogenic chemicals may raise ALL risk. **Down syndrome** and other inherited genetic conditions increase the risk of developing ALL in a person.

Immune System Disorders: Immune system-compromising conditions, like immunodeficiency disorders, may increase the risk of having ALL.

Symptoms: The signs and symptoms of ALL may resemble those of other forms of leukemia and may consist of:

- Weakness and Exhaustion
- Continual Infections
- Simple Bleeding or Bruising
- Joint or Bone Pain or Fever
- Enlarged lymph nodes
- Enlarged spleen or liver
- Appetite Loss and Weight Loss

★ **Diagnosis**:

The following examinations and techniques are frequently used to identify ALL:

Complete blood counts (CBCs) are blood tests used to determine the quantity and diversity of blood cells.

Bone marrow aspiration and biopsy: To check for the presence of leukemic cells in the bone marrow cells.

Cytogenetic analysis is the process of examining leukemic cells to find specific chromosomal abnormalities.

Lumbar Puncture: To examine the cerebrospinal fluid that surrounds the brain and spinal cord for leukemia cells.

★ **Treatment**

ALL is often treated aggressively with the goal of achieving remission (the absence of identifiable cancer cells). The main forms of treatment are:

Chemotherapy: The cornerstone of ALL treatment, which uses anticancer medications to destroy leukemia cells. To stop the spread of leukemia cells, radiation therapy is occasionally used to target certain regions, such as the brain and spinal cord.

Stem cell transplantation: In some situations, a peripheral blood or bone marrow stem cell transplant may be recommended, particularly for high-risk or relapsed cases.

Targeted therapy: In some circumstances, leukemia cells may be treated with specific medications that target particular proteins or genetic abnormalities.

Immunotherapy: To assist the immune system in locating and eliminating leukemia cells, certain patients may receive immunotherapy.

Age, general health, and genetic anomalies are a few different factors that can affect the prognosis for ALL. The prognosis for ALL in children and adults has dramatically improved thanks to therapy advances. Many patients have a chance of being cured with the current medicines and have long-term remission.

In order to identify and treat any potential relapses or late side effects of treatment, regular follow-up and monitoring are crucial. To improve their treatment outcomes and quality of life, patients with ALL require ongoing support and care from a multidisciplinary team that includes oncologists, hematologists, and supportive care specialists.

➢ Acute Myeloid Leukemia (AML)

The cancerous condition known as acute myeloid leukemia (AML) affects the bone marrow and blood and causes aberrant myeloid cells to multiply quickly.

The aberrant myeloid cells in AML do not mature properly and build up in the bone marrow and blood, in contrast to normal myeloid cells, which mature into red blood cells, platelets, and specific types of white blood cells. AML is more frequently diagnosed in adults, while it can affect anyone at any age. It is a somewhat aggressive type of leukemia that necessitates quick and thorough treatment. AML's precise etiology is frequently unknown, however a number of risk factors, such as the following, may raise the possibility of getting this form of leukemia:

Age: As people get older, their risk of developing AML rises.

Previous Cancer Treatment: Especially in the case of secondary AML, exposure to specific chemotherapy medications and radiation therapy used to treat other cancers can increase the chance of acquiring AML. Some people who have one of the blood illnesses known as **myelodysplastic syndromes** (MDS) are more likely to acquire AML.

Genetic Disorders: Down syndrome is one genetic abnormality that is linked to an increased chance of developing AML.

Smoking: Smoking cigarettes has been associated with a higher chance of acquiring AML.

The signs and symptoms of AML can change and change quickly over a short time. Typical warning signs and symptoms include:

- Weakness and Exhaustion
- Continual Infections
- Simple Bleeding or Bruising
- Paleness
- Breathlessness Joint pain or bone pain

- Enlarged lymph nodes
- Enlarged spleen or liver
- Unexplained Loss of weight
- Fever

★ Diagnosis

AML is diagnosed using a variety of tests and methods, which include:

<u>Complete blood counts</u> (CBCs) are blood tests used to determine the quantity and diversity of blood cells.

<u>Bone marrow aspiration and biopsy</u>: To check for the presence of leukemia cells in the bone marrow cells.

<u>Cytogenetic Analysis</u>: Detecting particular chromosomal abnormalities in leukemia cells.

<u>Flow Cytometry</u>: A method for examining the features of leukemia cells.

★ Treatment.

Remission, where there are no signs of leukemia cells in the bone marrow or blood, is the goal of AML treatment. The main forms of treatment are:

<u>Chemotherapy</u>: Intense chemotherapy, which uses potent medications to kill leukemia cells, is often used to treat AML.

<u>Stem cell transplantation</u>: For some patients, especially in high-risk or recurrent cases, a stem cell transplant (bone marrow or peripheral blood) may be advised.

Targeted Therapy: In some circumstances, it may be necessary to utilize medications that selectively target specific proteins on leukemia cells.

Supportive Care: While a patient is receiving treatment, supportive care techniques are used to control side effects, stop infections, and promote overall well being.

AML prognosis: The prognosis for AML is based on the patient's age, general health, and response to treatment, as well as the subtype of AML. Many patients' prospects have improved as a result of advancements in medicine, however individual prognosis might differ greatly.

For the purpose of identifying and managing any relapses or treatment-related problems, routine follow-up and monitoring are essential. To maximize their treatment success and quality of life, patients with AML require comprehensive care from a team of medical specialists, including oncologists, hematologists, and supportive care providers.

Chapter 4

Chronic Leukemia

➤ **Chronic Lymphocytic Leukaemia (CLL)**

A kind of cancer known as chronic lymphocytic leukemia (CLL) affects lymphocytes, which are white blood cells. In the bone marrow, blood, and lymph nodes, aberrant and mature lymphocytes gradually build up, which is how it is identified. The most prevalent form of adult leukemia is CLL, which usually affects older people. The typical age of diagnosis is around 70 years old.

Causes and Risk Factors

Although the specific cause of CLL is unknown, a number of things can raise your risk of getting it, including:

Age: Older persons are more likely to develop CLL, and the risk rises with age.

Family history: There may be a minor risk increase if CLL or other blood malignancies run in the family.

Genetic Predisposition: Particular genetic mutations might contribute to the emergence of CLL.

Long-Term Chemical Exposure: Long-term chemical exposure, including exposure to Agent Orange, may increase the risk of CLL.

Gender: Men are more likely than women to get CLL.

<u>**Symptoms**</u>

In its early stages, CLL may not manifest any symptoms at all, and it is frequently found by chance during normal blood tests. Common signs and symptoms of the condition include:

- Weakness and Exhaustion
- Increasing Infections in the Liver, Spleen, or Enlarged Lymph Nodes
- Evening sweats
- Unwanted Loss of Weight
- Simple Bleeding or Bruising
- Numerous nosebleeds

<u>**Diagnosis**</u>

Diagnosed by standard blood testing or by looking into symptoms connected to aberrant blood cell counts, CLL is frequently found. For diagnosis, the following examinations and techniques are used:

<u>Complete Blood Count (CBC)</u>: To determine the quantity and different blood cell types, including lymphocytes.

<u>Flow Cytometry</u>: This is a laboratory test which examines the properties of lymphocytes to see if they are abnormal.

<u>Bone marrow Aspiration and biopsy</u>: To look for aberrant cells in the bone marrow.

<u>Cytogenetic and Molecular testing</u>: Used in identifying certain genetic defects or mutations that may help inform treatment choices.

<u>**Treatment:**</u>

The course of CLL is largely determined by the disease's stage, its rate of progression, and the patient's general condition. Early-stage CLL may occasionally only need attentive monitoring and not urgent therapy. Options for treatment include:

<u>Chemotherapy</u>: Drugs that are typically used in chemotherapy may be utilized to kill cancer cells.

<u>Targeted Therapy</u>: Compared to conventional chemotherapy, specific medications that target particular proteins or metabolic processes in CLL cells may be employed.

<u>Immunotherapy</u>: The immune system can be assisted in locating and eliminating leukemia cells by the use of monoclonal antibodies or other immune-stimulating medications.

<u>Stem cell transplant</u>: Younger patients or those with high-risk diseases may occasionally be candidates for a stem cell transplant.

The prognosis for CLL varies greatly based on a number of variables, such as the stage and kind of the disease, genetic markers, age, and general health. While some CLL patients may experience a reasonably stable course of their disease and not need immediate treatment, others may experience disease progression and need continuing care.

To effectively manage CLL and provide appropriate treatment throughout the disease's course, regular monitoring and follow-up with medical professionals are crucial. Hematologists, oncologists, and supportive care professionals work together to provide comprehensive treatment for CLL patients in order to address both the physical and psychological effects of having leukemia.

> ### ➢ Chronic Myeloid Leukaemia (CML)

Specifically the myeloid cells, which give rise to red blood cells, platelets, and specific types of white blood cells, are affected by Chronic Myeloid Leukaemia (CML), a type of malignancy that affects the bone marrow and blood. In CML, the bone marrow experiences an abnormal and unchecked proliferation of immature myeloid cells (blasts), which causes an increase in the quantity of these abnormal cells in the blood.

Comparatively uncommon to other forms of leukemia, CML is more frequently found in adults and is diagnosed at an average age of roughly 60. There are three distinct phases that define it:

- Chronic Phase: The majority of patients are in the chronic phase at the time of diagnosis, which is typically slow-growing and may not produce noticeable symptoms.
- Accelerated Phase: In a few instances, CML can advance to an accelerated phase, in which the illness worsens and there are more blasts in the blood and bone marrow.
- Blast Crisis: CML can advance to the acute leukemia-like blast crisis stage if untreated or if the condition does not improve with treatment. Similar to acute myeloid leukemia (AML), this phase is marked by a significant rise in immature blast cells.

Chapter 5

Causes and Risk Factors

It's not always clear what causes leukemia, such as acute lymphocytic leukemia (ALL), acute myeloid leukemia (AML), chronic lymphocytic leukemia (CLL), and chronic myeloid leukemia (CML). There are, however, a number of risk factors that may raise the possibility of these leukemias manifesting. It's crucial to remember that having one or more risk factors is not a guarantee that leukemia will develop, and that many people who have the disease have no discernible risk factors. The following are some typical causes and risk factors:

Genetic Propensity: Leukaemia may occasionally arise due to specific genetic mutations or chromosomal abnormalities. For instance, there can be particular genetic alterations, like the Philadelphia chromosome in CML or the presence of particular genes linked to a higher risk of leukemia.

Age: Older people are more likely to develop leukemia, especially AML and CLL. However, children and young adults are more frequently diagnosed with ALL.

Radiation Exposure: A higher incidence of leukemia has been linked to high levels of ionizing radiation exposure. People who have had radiation therapy for prior cancers or who have been exposed to nuclear accidents should pay particular attention to this.

Chemical Exposure: Leukaemia risk may be increased by exposure to some carcinogenic chemicals, including benzene and some industrial chemicals.

Prior cancer therapies: Some chemotherapy medicines, especially those used to treat secondary leukemia, may make it more likely for people to acquire leukemia. It's important to remember that, in most cases, the advantages of receiving cancer therapy outweigh the potential hazards of contracting leukemia.

Family History: Having a leukemia or other blood condition in the family may marginally raise your risk of getting the disease. Children with Fanconi anemia and certain other genetic diseases, such as Down syndrome, are more likely to acquire leukemia than other children.

Gender: Males are more likely to develop some kinds of leukemia, such as CLL and AML.

Viral Infections: Leukaemia risk has been associated with some viral infections, including human T-cell leukemia virus (HTLV-1), Epstein-Barr virus (EBV), and human immunodeficiency virus (HIV).

Immune System Disorders: Some immune system problems or illnesses that compromise the immune system may raise the chance of leukemia development. It is crucial to realize that while these risk factors may be linked to a higher chance of acquiring leukemia, the majority of leukemia cases lack a clear-cut etiology. The fundamental mechanisms and contributing variables for the various kinds of leukemia are still being studied. In order to manage and improve the results for those who have been diagnosed with leukemia, early detection and prompt treatment are still essential. It is best to speak with a healthcare professional for individualized advice and recommendations if you are worried about your chance of acquiring leukemia or any other health problem.

Chapter 6

Symptoms

➤ **General Signs and Symptoms**

In the early stages of the disease, leukemia, including acute lymphoblastic leukemia (ALL), acute myeloid leukemia (AML), chronic lymphocytic leukemia (CLL), and chronic myeloid leukemia (CML), share certain common basic symptoms. Depending on the type and stage of the leukemia, these symptoms may differ in their severity and presentation. Common general signs and symptoms include:

<u>Weakness and Fatigue:</u> Leukaemia frequently manifests as persistent, inexplicable fatigue or a sense of weakness. It frequently results from a decline in healthy blood cells, which lowers the blood's ability to carry oxygen.

<u>Frequent Infections</u>: Leukaemia can affect an individual's immune system's ability to operate normally, leaving them more prone to infections. Patients may suffer from persistent or severe infections, such as skin, urinary tract, or respiratory infections.

<u>Easy Bruising or Bleeding:</u> Low platelet counts (thrombocytopenia) brought on by leukemia can cause nosebleeds, easy bruising, and protracted bleeding from small cuts or wounds.

<u>Pallor:</u> A reduction in red blood cells (anemia) can make the skin and mucous membranes seem pale and devoid of a healthy color.

Unexpected and unplanned weight loss: This may happen if you have leukemia, especially if the disease is advanced.

Joint or Bone discomfort: Leukaemia can result in joint or bone discomfort, particularly in the hips and sternum. This discomfort is brought on by the bone marrow swelling brought on by an overabundance of aberrant cells.

Swollen Lymph Nodes: Leukaemia symptoms may include swollen lymph nodes, particularly those in the neck, armpits, or groin.

Spleen or Liver Enlargement: The liver and spleen may increase as a result of an accumulation of leukemia cells. The effect could be bloating or discomfort in the abdomen.

Night Sweats: Excessive sweating, particularly while sleeping, is a frequent symptom, especially in leukemia that has advanced stages.

Fever: Some people with leukemia may have recurring or persistent fevers that have no apparent reason.

It's crucial to keep in mind that these symptoms can be brought on by a variety of diseases, so just because you have one or more of them doesn't mean you have leukemia. To ensure a complete evaluation and diagnosis, you must see a healthcare professional if your symptoms persist or get worse. Effective leukemia management and better outcomes depend on early detection and prompt treatment.

➢ **Specific signs of different types of leukemia**

Depending on the type of leukemia and the blood cells involved, specific symptoms for various types of leukemia can change. The precise symptoms linked to each kind are listed below:

Acute Lymphocytic Leukaemia (ALL)

- Weakness and Exhaustion
- Continual Infections
- Simple Bleeding or Bruising Paleness
- Bone or joint pain, enlarged lymph nodes, liver, or spleen
- Fever

In situations where leukemia cells move to the central nervous system, headaches and vision issues may occur.

Leukaemia Acute Myeloid (AML):

- Weakness and Exhaustion
- Continual Infections
- Simple Bleeding or Bruising Paleness
- Joint or bone pain, enlarged liver, spleen, or fever
- Numerous nosebleeds
- Bleeding Gums

Acute Myeloid Leukaemia (AML):

- Weakness and Exhaustion
- Frequent Infections with Enlarged Lymph Nodes, Liver, or Spleen
- Simple Bleeding or Bruising Night Sweats
- Unwanted Loss of Weight

- Repeated Fever

Chronic Myeloid Leukaemia (CML)

- Weakness and Exhaustion
- Spleen Enlargement (Splenomegaly)
- Discomfort or fullness in the Abdomen
- Unwanted Loss of Weight
- Evening sweats
- Fever
- Joint pain and Bone pain
- Simple Bleeding or Bruising
- Multiple Infections

It's critical to remember that these symptoms might differ in severity and presentation for every person, and some leukemia patients may not experience all of them. Additionally, other medical problems can also induce these symptoms, thus they are not just related to leukemia. It is crucial to speak with a healthcare expert for an accurate examination, diagnosis, and management if you encounter any recurring or alarming symptoms. Effective leukemia management and better outcomes depend on early detection and prompt treatment.

Chapter 7

Diagnosis

1. <u>Laboratory evaluations and blood testing</u>

Leukaemia and other medical disorders must be diagnosed and monitored with the help of blood testing and laboratory analysis. These tests aid medical specialists in assessing the quantity and makeup of blood cells, spotting any abnormal ones, and figuring out the subtype and stage of leukemia. Key blood tests and laboratory analysis utilized in the assessment of leukemia include the following:

→ One of the most popular blood tests to determine the general state of the blood and the presence of abnormalities is the complete blood count (CBC). The following information is provided by a CBC:

→ Measures of hemoglobin, hematocrit, and red blood cell count are among the red blood cells (RBC) tests that can assist to determine an individual's ability to carry oxygen and identify anemia.

→ Counts of several types of white blood cells, such as neutrophils, lymphocytes, monocytes, eosinophils, and basophils, are included in the category of white blood cells (WBC). Leukaemia or infections may be indicated by abnormal WBC levels.

→ Low platelet counts can cause easy bleeding or bruising. Platelets: The platelet count is crucial for determining how well blood clots.

→ Peripheral Blood Smear: To make a blood smear, put a drop of blood on a glass slide, use special chemicals to stain it, and then examine the smear under a microscope. It enables the assessment of blood cell shape and aids in the identification of aberrant cells, such as blasts or atypical lymphocytes, which might be an indication of leukemia.

→ Bone Marrow Aspiration and Biopsy: These techniques are used to collect a sample of the bone marrow and the surrounding bone for analysis. These tests assist examine the general health of the bone marrow and calculate the percentage of blasts or aberrant cells in the bone marrow.

→ Cytogenetic analysis: In order to detect any specific genetic abnormalities, such as the Philadelphia chromosome in Chronic Myeloid Leukaemia (CML), cytogenetic testing examines the chromosomes in leukemia cells. Determining the leukemia subtype and making treatment decisions require this information.

→ Molecular testing: Molecular testing enables the detection of particular genetic fusions or mutations that may exist in leukemia cells. BCR-ABL1 testing, for instance, is used to identify and track CML.

→ Flow cytometry is a method used to examine the features of individual cells, including their size, shape, and particular surface markers. It is useful for locating and describing aberrant leukemia cells.

→ Spinal tap or lumbar puncture may be used in specific circumstances to remove cerebrospinal fluid from the spinal canal for testing. If leukemia cells have reached the central nervous system, this treatment can help identify that.

Along with other diagnostic techniques, these blood tests and laboratory analysis aid medical practitioners in correctly diagnosing leukemia, identifying its subtype and stage, and formulating effective treatment plans. Blood counts and other test indicators must be regularly monitored in order to assess therapy effectiveness and spot any illness progression or relapse.

2.   <u>Aspiration and biopsy of the bone marrow</u>

Important diagnostic techniques used to assess the bone marrow, which is the soft, spongy substance found inside bones, include bone marrow biopsy and bone marrow aspiration. Leukaemia and other blood disorders are assessed using these methods often. They offer important details on the condition and make-up of the bone marrow, including the quantity and variety of blood cells produced as well as the presence of aberrant cells.

- ➔ Bone Marrow Aspiration: A tiny sample of liquid bone marrow is taken from the bone using a thin, hollow needle during a bone marrow aspiration. The posterior iliac crest on the back of the hipbone and, less frequently, the sternum (breastbone) are the two most frequent locations for bone marrow aspiration. To reduce pain, the treatment is often carried out under local anesthetic.

- ➔ Blood cells of all types, including platelets, white blood cells, red blood cells, and immature blood cells known as blasts, can be found in the liquid bone marrow sample taken by aspiration. The diagnosis and classification of leukemia can be greatly aided by abnormalities in the quantity or characteristics of blasts in the bone marrow.

→ Bone Marrow Biopsy: In addition to a bone marrow aspiration, a bone marrow biopsy is frequently carried out. A somewhat larger needle is used in a bone marrow biopsy to take a larger sample of bone marrow and a small piece of the nearby bone. The biopsy sample is subsequently delivered to a lab for analysis.

The results of the bone marrow biopsy include details regarding the cellular makeup and general structure of the bone marrow. It aids in determining the distribution of different cell types as well as any alterations or anomalies in the structure of the bone marrow. An important factor in correctly identifying and staging leukemia is the presence and location of aberrant cells, which can be shown by a bone marrow biopsy.

Both bone marrow aspiration and biopsy are crucial steps in the leukemia diagnosis procedure. The majority of these operations are risk-free, and any discomfort that may be felt during them is usually mild and easily handled. Patients may suffer slight pain at the biopsy site after the operations, but this often goes away soon.

Pathologists and hematologists carefully scrutinize the bone marrow samples obtained during aspiration and biopsy because they are crucial to the diagnosis and characterization of leukemia and other blood diseases. The data gathered from these procedures aids in directing therapy choices and continuing illness monitoring.

3.   <u>Cytogenetic analysis and molecular testing</u>

Cytogenetic analysis and molecular testing are laboratory techniques used to study the genetic characteristics of cells, particularly in the context of cancer and blood disorders like leukemia. These tests are crucial in the diagnosis, classification, and management of leukemia, as they provide valuable information about specific genetic abnormalities and mutations present in leukemia cells. Here's a brief overview of cytogenetic analysis and molecular testing:

→ <u>Cytogenetic Analysis:</u> Cytogenetic analysis involves the study of the chromosomal structure and abnormalities in cells, particularly cancer cells. In leukemia, specific chromosomal abnormalities can play a significant role in the development and progression of the disease. Cytogenetic analysis helps identify these abnormalities, which can aid in determining the subtype of leukemia and predicting its clinical behavior. In this test, leukemia cells from a bone marrow sample are cultured and treated to arrest them at the metaphase stage of cell division. The chromosomes are then stained and examined under a microscope to visualize their structure. Abnormalities, such as translocations (exchange of genetic material between chromosomes), deletions, or other rearrangements, can be detected and identified. For example, the presence of the Philadelphia chromosome in Chronic Myeloid Leukaemia (CML) is detected through cytogenetic analysis.

→ <u>Molecular Testing:</u> Molecular testing involves analyzing the genetic material (DNA or RNA) of cells to detect specific mutations or genetic alterations. This type of testing is highly sensitive and can identify changes at the molecular level, even when cytogenetic analysis may not reveal visible chromosomal abnormalities. In leukemia, molecular testing is often used to identify fusion genes and mutations that are characteristic of certain leukemia subtypes. For example, in Chronic Myeloid Leukaemia (CML), molecular testing is used to detect the BCR-ABL1 fusion gene, which results from the Philadelphia chromosome abnormality. Molecular testing can also be used to monitor the response to treatment and detect minimal residual disease (MRD) in some leukemia cases. The results of cytogenetic analysis and molecular testing play a crucial role in guiding treatment decisions and assessing the prognosis for individuals with leukemia. Specific genetic abnormalities can influence the choice of targeted therapies and help healthcare providers predict the patient's response to treatment.

Both cytogenetic analysis and molecular testing require specialized laboratories and expertise. They are essential components of the comprehensive diagnostic approach used to characterize leukemia and provide personalized treatment strategies for each patient. These tests are typically performed on bone marrow or blood samples obtained from patients during the diagnostic workup and throughout the course of treatment to monitor disease progression and response to therapy.

Chapter 8

Treatment

<u>Chemotherapy</u>

Chemotherapy is a type of cancer treatment that employs potent medications to either kill or stop rapidly dividing cells, especially cancer cells, from proliferating and replicating. It is one of the main forms of treatment for many cancers, including leukemia. Chemotherapy can be given orally as pills, intravenously (IV) as an infusion, or intramuscularly (IM) as an injection.

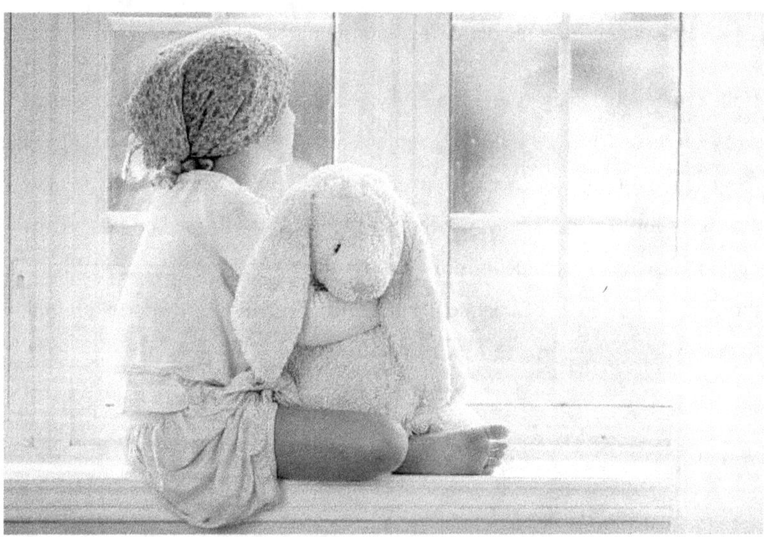

Chemotherapy medications target cells that are aggressively dividing, which is a trait of cancer cells. This is how chemotherapy works. However, because some of the body's healthy, normal cells divide quickly, chemotherapy can also have an adverse effect on these cells. Chemotherapy aims to specifically target and kill cancer cells while causing the least amount of harm to healthy cells.

Chemotherapy is used to treat a variety of leukemias, including acute lymphoblastic leukemia (ALL), acute myeloid leukemia (AML), chronic lymphocytic leukemia (CLL), and some forms of chronic myeloid leukemia (CML). Depending on the kind of leukemia, the patient's age, general health, and other considerations, different chemotherapy medications, dosages, and treatment regimens are used.

Chemotherapy is often administered as part of vigorous and rigorous treatment plans known as induction therapy for acute leukemias (ALL and AML). Remission, in which there are no identifiable leukemia cells in the bone marrow or blood, is the desired outcome of induction therapy. In order to eradicate as many leukemia cells as possible, high doses of chemotherapy medications are given during a brief period of time. To further lower the chance of disease recurrence, consolidation therapy and maintenance therapy may be given after induction therapy.

Chemotherapy may be used as part of the treatment strategy for chronic leukemias (CLL and CML), however it is frequently supplemented with other targeted medicines. Combining monoclonal antibodies (such as rituximab) with chemotherapeutic medications like fludarabine and cyclophosphamide may be used to treat CLL. Tyrosine kinase inhibitors (TKIs) are the mainstay of targeted therapy for CML, while chemotherapy may also be employed in some cases or in combination with TKIs for particular patients. Chemotherapy's impact on the body's rapidly dividing healthy cells, including those in the bone marrow, hair follicles, digestive system, and mouth, might result in adverse effects.

Chemotherapy frequently has adverse consequences like:

- Fatigue
- Nausea and diarrhea
- Hair fall
- Decreased blood cell counts, which can cause anemia and raise the risk of bleeding and infection
- Oral sores
- Reduced appetite
- Constipation or diarrhea

These adverse effects are typically transient and can be controlled with supportive care drugs and dietary changes. Throughout chemotherapy, the medical staff keeps a constant eye on the patients to manage side effects and guarantee the greatest results.

Chemotherapy is still a crucial part of treating leukemia, and research is always being done to increase its efficacy while lowering its negative effects. Depending on the features of each patient as well as the precise subtype and stage of their leukemia, treatment recommendations are made.

Radiation Therapy

High-energy radiation is used in radiation therapy, sometimes referred to as radiotherapy, as a cancer treatment to target and kill cancer cells or halt their growth. It is frequently used to treat many cancers, including leukemia. Radiation therapy is a localized treatment that concentrates on specific locations where cancer cells are present, in contrast to chemotherapy, which treats the entire body through the bloodstream.

Radiation therapy interferes with cancer cells' capacity to grow and divide by damaging the DNA within those cells. This causes the cancer cells to die either directly or indirectly stopping them from proliferating. Radiation can also harm healthy normal cells, but they typically have a higher capacity for self-healing than cancer cells. Radiation therapy's objective is to deliver just the right amount of radiation to the cancer cells while preserving as much of the surrounding healthy tissue as feasible.

Radiation therapy comes in two main varieties, both of which are used to treat leukemia:

❖ External Beam Radiation Therapy (EBRT): Radiation is delivered from outside the body using a device known as a linear accelerator. The system precisely directs radiation beams at the desired location, such as the leukemia-affected bone marrow or lymph nodes, while the patient is lying on a treatment table. Usually, the treatment is given over a number of sessions (fractions) spaced out over several weeks.

❖ Total Body Irradiation (TBI) is a specific type of radiation therapy that exposes the entire body to radiation. In the treatment of some cases of acute myeloid leukemia (AML) and acute lymphocytic leukemia (ALL), it is frequently used as a component of the regimen prior to stem cell or bone marrow transplantation. In order to improve the engraftment of donor cells during the transplant operation, TBI is utilized to destroy cancer cells and suppress the immune system.

Radiation therapy is not frequently utilized as the main leukemia treatment, however it may be used in some circumstances, such as:

- Localized Disease: Radiation therapy may be utilized to treat leukemia in some circumstances, such as when the disease has only affected a single lymph node or an extramedullary location. Radiation therapy can be used as palliative care when leukemia has spread to a specific area and is causing pain or discomfort in order to reduce symptoms and enhance quality of life.

- Pre-Transplant Conditioning: As was already noted, some leukemia patients may benefit from Total Body Irradiation as a part of their pre-transplant program before receiving a stem cell or bone marrow transplant.

Radiation therapy side effects: Radiation therapy side effects are influenced by the area being treated and the radiation dose administered. Typical negative effects include:

- Fatigue
- Skin modifications in the treated area (redness, itchiness, and dryness in the treated region)
- Hair loss
- Nausea or vomiting
- Low levels of red blood cells (if radiation damages bone marrow)

The majority of radiation therapy side effects are transient and go away after the course of treatments. The radiation oncology team carefully prepares the course of treatment to reduce side effects and offer comfort care while the therapy is being administered.

Overall, the use of radiation therapy depends on the exact type, stage, and location of the disease, as well as the patient's overall health and treatment objectives. Radiation therapy is a significant treatment option in some cases of leukemia. To provide the patient with the best outcome possible, the healthcare team collaborates to create a thorough treatment plan that may include radiation therapy, chemotherapy, targeted therapies, and other modalities.

Targeted Therapy

Leukaemia treatment, like other cancer treatments, must include supportive care and symptom control. Throughout the course of the disease, these supportive measures are intended to improve the patient's general health, control treatment-related side effects, and improve quality of life. Along with the primary cancer therapy, supportive care is offered, and it is customized to meet the needs of each patient. Key components of supportive treatment and symptom control in leukemia include the following:

★ Pain management: Pain is a frequent sign of leukemia, particularly when the bone marrow is affected. Utilizing medicines, physical therapy, and other interventions to reduce pain and increase comfort is part of effective pain management.

★ Chemotherapy and other cancer treatments can make you feel sick to your stomach and make you vomit. Antiemetic drugs are administered to patients to help them tolerate their therapies better and prevent or lessen these side effects.

★ <u>Managing Fatigue:</u> A common symptom of leukemia, fatigue can have a substantial influence on a patient's quality of life and daily activities. Fatigue can be controlled with enough sleep, a healthy diet, and little exercise. Severe weariness may occasionally be treated with medicine.

★ <u>Preventing Infections</u>: Patients with leukemia are more susceptible to infections because the disease affects their immune system and because of the side effects of therapies like chemotherapy. To lower the risk of infections, preventive steps are crucial, such as vaccines and avoiding contact with sick people.

★ <u>Transfusions of blood:</u> Leukaemia and its therapies can cause low blood cell counts, which can cause anemia, low platelet counts, and weakened immunity. Platelets and packed red blood cells can be given as part of blood transfusions to make up for these shortages and enhance health.

★ <u>Support for adequate nutrition</u>: It's important for leukemia patients to maintain good nutrition. A dietician can assist in developing a healthy meal plan that takes the patient's unique needs into consideration and tackles any eating difficulties that may develop throughout therapy.

★ <u>Psychological and Emotional Support</u>: Receiving a leukemia diagnosis can be emotionally taxing for both the sufferer and their loved ones. People can manage stress, anxiety, and depression by getting counseling, joining support groups, and undergoing psychological interventions.

★ <u>Treatment for Mucositis and Dental Care:</u> Chemotherapy and radiation treatment can cause mucositis, an inflammation of the mouth and throat. The risk of infections can be decreased and discomfort can be reduced with proper dental care and pain management.

★ <u>Addressing Sleep Disturbances:</u> Leukaemia treatments and sleep habits can both be affected. To manage sleep disruptions, approaches for good sleep hygiene, relaxation exercises, and pharmaceuticals may be employed.

★ <u>Care</u>: Palliative care aims to enhance the quality of life for patients who are suffering from life-threatening conditions, such as leukemia. It can be given at any stage of the disease and takes care of requirements on the bodily, emotional, and spiritual levels.

Comprehensive cancer care must include both symptom control and supportive care. To provide individualized supportive care based on the patient's particular requirements and preferences, a multidisciplinary team of healthcare professionals; including oncologists, nurses, palliative care experts, social workers, and others, works together. Throughout their cancer journey, the patient's comfort and wellbeing should be prioritized.

Chapter 9

Prognosis and Survival Rates

A. **Factors influencing prognosis**

The prognosis for leukemia, like any other cancer, is impacted by a number of variables that aid medical professionals in anticipating the likely course of the illness and the likelihood of successful therapy. Depending on the type of leukemia, the patient's general condition, and the illness stage, these variables may change. The following are some of the major elements affecting the leukemia prognosis:

→ Leukaemia Subtype: The prognosis for various leukemia subtypes varies. While certain forms of leukemia are more aggressive and challenging to treat, others respond better to medication. For instance, compared to acute myeloid leukemia (AML) in older individuals, acute lymphocytic leukemia (ALL) in youngsters typically has a greater cure rate.

→ Disease Stage: The prognosis is greatly influenced by the leukemia's stage at the time of diagnosis. The prognosis for early-stage leukemia, which is localized or restricted to a single location, is often better than for advanced-stage leukemia, which has spread to numerous organs or distant sites.

→ Genetic and molecular markers: The behavior of the disease and how it responds to treatment can be influenced by certain genetic abnormalities or mutations in leukemia cells. For instance, Chronic Myeloid Leukaemia (CML) with the Philadelphia chromosome has a worse prognosis without targeted therapy.

→ Age: Leukaemia prognosis is significantly impacted by age. Because they can withstand more extensive therapies and are better able to recover from therapy-related side effects, children and younger adults frequently have better outcomes than older adults.

→ Overall Health and Fitness: A patient's capacity to tolerate therapy and recover from side effects might be affected by their overall health and fitness level. The prognosis for those with additional underlying medical issues could be worse.

→ Response to treatments: An important determinant of prognosis is how well the leukemia responds to the early treatments (induction therapy). A better prognosis is linked to a complete remission (absence of detectable leukemia cells) following induction therapy.

→ Minimal Residual Disease (MRD): A few leukemia cells may still be present in trace amounts in the bone marrow or blood even after remission. Sensitive diagnostic techniques for MRD detection can affect prognosis and direct future treatment choices. The prognosis for some high-risk leukemia cases can be greatly impacted by getting a stem cell transplant (bone marrow transplant) from a compatible donor, even direct siblings.

→ Supportive Care and Complication Management: Complications and infections caused by the treatment have an impact on the prognosis as a whole.

The prognosis for each person varies, and there are no two leukemia cases that are exactly comparable. The exact course of a patient's disease cannot be predicted by prognostic variables, but they can aid in informing treatment choices and providing an estimate of outcomes. These elements are used by healthcare professionals to create a thorough treatment plan that offers the greatest potential for success while taking the patient's unique situation and preferences into account.

B. Survival rates for various leukemia kinds and stages

Based on a number of variables, including the kind of leukemia, the patient's age, the stage at diagnosis, and the accessibility and efficacy of treatment choices, survival rates for various types and stages of leukemia might fluctuate dramatically. The percentage of people who are still living five years after their diagnosis is the conventional basis that survival rates are stated. It is significant to remember that survival rates are statistical estimates and do not indicate how a particular patient will fare. Following are some average survival rates for various leukemia kinds and stages:

➢ ALL: Acute lymphocytic leukemia

Children with ALL have a five-year survival rate of 90% or higher overall. Pediatric ALL survival rates have greatly increased as a result of therapy advancements.Adults with ALL typically have a poorer five-year survival rate, between 30% and 40%. Adults ALL frequently exhibit greater aggression and less therapeutic response.

➢ Acute Myeloid Leukaemia (AML)

Age and cytogenetic/molecular features, as well as other variables, affect the overall five-year survival rate for AML. The average five-year survival rate for AML is typically between 25% and 30%. Younger patients and those who qualify for extensive therapies have higher survival rates.

➢ Chronic Lymphocytic Leukaemia (CLL)

CLL is a leukemia that advances quite slowly. CLL has a five-year overall survival rate of 85% to 90%. Many CLL patients progress slowly and may not need immediate therapy.

> ➤ **Chronic Myeloid Leukaemia (CML)**

The prognosis for CML has significantly improved since tyrosine kinase inhibitor (TKI) therapy was introduced. Today, the overall CML five-year survival rate is higher than 90%. With continuous targeted therapy, many patients experience prolonged profound remissions and can resume their normal lives.

It is critical to keep in mind that survival rates are calculated using information from large patient populations and do not account for individual variances. Age, general health, particular genetic variations, treatment response, and access to healthcare are just a few examples of the variables that might affect a person's prognosis. Additionally, continuous studies and improvements in leukemia therapies continue to increase patient survival rates and quality of life. For a personalized evaluation and comprehension of their leukemia prognosis, patients should talk with their healthcare provider about their particular prognosis and treatment options.

Chapter 10
Support and Coping

Effects on patients' and relatives' mental health

Leukemia diagnoses and the ensuing course of therapy can have a significant psychological impact on patients and their families. Leukaemia is a serious, life-threatening condition that can cause a wide range of emotions and difficulties, some of which may last the duration of the cancer journey. The following are some typical psychological effects on patients and families:

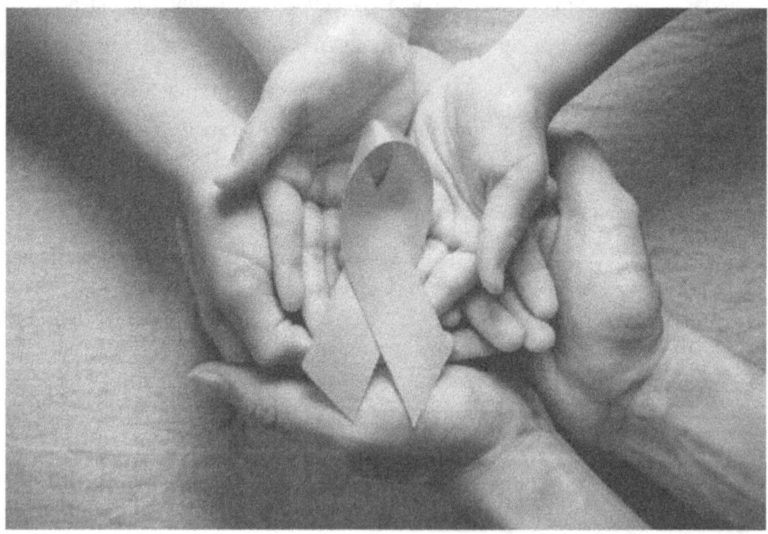

* <u>Dread and Anxiety</u>: The initial shock of the diagnosis and the unknowns around the future might cause dread and anxiety. Patients may be

concerned about their prognosis, the results of their treatment, and possible therapy side effects.

* ❖ <u>Depression and Sadness:</u> Coping with a cancer diagnosis and the difficulties of treatment might result in depressive and saddening sentiments. It can be extremely difficult to deal with the disease's physical and psychological effects.
* ❖ <u>Stress and Uncertainty</u>: Leukaemia treatment entails a number of doctor visits, tests, and procedures. Both patients and their family may experience stress due to the unknown nature of the disease and the course of treatment.
* ❖ <u>Grief and Loss</u>: Receiving a leukemia diagnosis can make patients feel like they have lost something, particularly if they are unable to continue with past hobbies or undergo bodily changes as a result of treatment.
* ❖ <u>Impact on Family Dynamics</u>: A leukemia diagnosis can have a big impact on family dynamics. To help the patient during therapy, family members may need to assume new roles and duties.
* ❖ <u>Financial worries</u>: The high cost of leukemia treatment might cause financial strain and fear about upcoming medical costs.
* ❖ <u>Body Image and Self-Esteem</u>: Physical changes brought on by treatment, such as hair loss, weight changes, and scarring, may have an effect on one's perception of one's body and self.

Coping with Treatment Side Effects

Patients may find it difficult to manage treatment-related side effects such nausea, exhaustion, and discomfort, which can have an impact on their emotional health. Leukaemia can cause relationships with partners, friends, and family to become strained. It may be difficult for patients and family members to appropriately express their sentiments and emotions.

Fear of Recurrence: Even after successful therapy and remission, there may still be persistent worries of leukemia returning, causing tension and worry.

Patients' and families' support

Comprehensive cancer care must include psychological assistance. To address their emotional needs and manage the difficulties of leukemia, patients and family should have access to counseling, support groups, and psychological services. Helping patients and families deal with the psychosocial effects of leukemia requires the support of medical doctors, social workers, and mental health specialists.

Fears and concerns can be addressed with the aid of open dialogue between family members and with medical professionals. Sharing experiences with people who have gone through comparable circumstances can also help to understand and support one another. Patients and family are urged to seek support and communicate their feelings because doing so can help them cope better with this trying period and feel better overall.

Counseling and Support Services

Support groups and counseling programs are essential for giving people and families dealing with leukemia and other cancer-related issues emotional support, knowledge, and coping mechanisms. These programs are intended to help patients and their loved ones deal with the psychological, emotional, and social elements of dealing with the condition. Here are a few typical forms of support that are available to people with leukemia and their families:

- ❖ Advisory Groups

<u>Leukemia-specific Support Groups</u>: Members of these groups must have received a leukemia diagnosis or be their caretakers. Sharing experiences, worries, and coping mechanisms fosters mutual understanding and support. Leukemia-specific support groups are available, but hospitals, cancer centers, and community organizations may also host general cancer support groups. These organizations bring together people with a range of cancer diagnoses to share experiences and offer support to one another.

- ❖ Individual therapy

Counselors with competence in offering emotional support and counseling to cancer patients and their families are known as psychosocial oncology counselors. They can assist people with managing stress, coping with the psychological effects of leukemia, and addressing issues with treatment and surviving.

<u>Oncology Social Workers</u>: Oncology social workers can connect patients and families with community services to help fulfill their needs, in addition to offering patients and families practical assistance and emotional support.

- ❖ Communities of Support Online

Patients and caregivers can interact with people going through similar circumstances, share stories, and get information from the comfort of their homes through online support groups and forums.

- ❖ Cancer centers or hospitals-based support programs

Support services designed to meet the needs of leukemia patients and their families are offered by many hospitals and cancer treatment facilities. Support groups, counseling services, educational courses, and wellness activities could all be a part of these programs.

❖ Workshops and webinars for education

Various elements of leukemia, treatment options, side effect management, and survivorship are covered in educational workshops and webinars that are provided by several organizations and cancer hospitals.

❖ Spiritual and Religious Support

Hospitals or nearby religious institutions may offer spiritual and religious support. In trying circumstances, chaplains and spiritual advisers can offer solace and assistance. People should look into various support options to determine which ones best meet their needs.

Participating in support groups and counseling can foster a sense of belonging, lessen feelings of loneliness, and offer helpful coping mechanisms for overcoming leukemia's obstacles. Patients and families are encouraged to address their emotional needs and concerns with their medical team since healthcare professionals may frequently provide information and recommendations to appropriate support resources.

Self-care and lifestyle adjustments during treatment

During leukemia treatment, lifestyle adjustments and self-care routines can dramatically improve a patient's health, treatment results, and general quality of life. Following are some significant dietary adjustments and self-care techniques that leukemia patients may think about while undergoing treatment:

- Nutrition:

In order to strengthen the body's immune system and keep one's strength during treatment, one must consume a healthy, balanced diet. A mix of fruits, vegetables, whole grains, lean proteins, and healthy fats should be included in a patient's diet.

A licensed dietitian can offer individualized advice and propose relevant dietary modifications if treatment-related side effects, such as mouth sores or nausea, affect eating habits.

- Hydration:

It's important to stay hydrated, especially when receiving chemotherapy or radiation treatment. Dehydration can be avoided and toxins can be removed from the body by drinking plenty of water.

- Physical Exercise:

Regular physical activity, if tolerated, can assist maintain muscle strength while reducing fatigue and improving mood. To assess the proper degree of exercise based on a person's health and treatment state, speak with the medical staff.

- Sleep and rest:

Healing and general well-being depend on getting enough sleep and rest. Patients should make obtaining enough sleep a priority and pay attention to their bodies' cues to rest when they need to.

- Stress Reduction:

During treatment, stress-reduction strategies like meditation, yoga, deep breathing exercises, or mindfulness exercises can help lower anxiety and enhance emotional wellbeing.

- Avoiding alcohol and smoking:

Alcohol abuse and smoking both have negative health implications, especially when undergoing cancer therapy. Patients are encouraged to minimize their alcohol consumption and quit smoking.

- Preventing Contact with Illness:

Due to their compromised immune systems, leukemia patients are more prone to infections. Infection risk can be lowered by taking steps to prevent contact with ill people and by using proper hand hygiene.

- Using Sunscreen:

Some medical procedures can make patients more sensitive to sunlight. Sunburn and skin damage can be avoided by using sunscreen and protective clothes.

- Emotional assistance:

An outlet for expressing emotions and worries can be found by seeking emotional assistance through counseling, support groups, or talking with close friends and family.

- Having conversations with the medical staff:

It's critical to be open with the medical staff about any adverse effects of the treatment, worries, and general wellbeing. The medical staff can advise and modify treatment regimens as necessary.

Patients must keep in mind that self-care techniques are unique and may change based on the particular treatment and individual health circumstances. Before beginning any new self-care routines or making any significant alterations to their way of life while receiving treatment for leukemia, patients should always get advice from their medical team. The medical staff can make tailored recommendations to accommodate each patient's particular demands and therapeutic journey.

Chapter 11

Current trends and intervention in the treatment of leukemia

When patients undergo allogeneic bone marrow transplantation (BMT) during the chronic phase of CML or the initial remission of AML and ALL, more than 50% of patients are cured. On the other hand, chemotherapeutic treatment for acute leukemia has made significant strides recently. About 40–50% of adults with AML undergoing intensive chemotherapy report disease-free survival (DFS) at three years. The use of BMT versus intensive chemotherapy in the treatment of AML has thus been the subject of numerous prospective randomized clinical trials. Significant differences in DFS were found only in a few studies though the results of BMT appear to be comparable or superior to chemotherapy.

Therefore, the overall advantage of BMT in first remission AML is smaller than expected.Instead of deciding whether to undertake chemotherapy or a transplant, we could decide whether to perform chemotherapy first and save the transplant for a last resort. All-trans retinoic acid has recently been used in differentiation therapy to successfully treat acute promyelocytic leukemia. Some patients with myelodysplastic syndrome and atypical AML have also been shown to respond well to low-dose aclarubicin when used as differentiation treatment. A number of cytokines are now usable in clinical settings thanks to advancements in their molecular biology.

As powerful inducers of granulocyte-macrophage production, G-CSF, GM-CSF, and M-CSF are excellent for speeding up the hematologic recovery following chemotherapy-induced myelosuppression or BMT. Several researches have employed interferon-alpha (IFN-alpha). Additionally, long-term IFN-alpha therapy can reduce Ph chromosomal positivity; in some individuals, Ph-positive clones may even be undetectable. Therefore, even if BMT is intended, IFN-alpha will be the preferred form of treatment for CML.

Chapter 12

Conclusion

→ Recap of Leukaemia and its Impact

A form of cancer known as leukemia affects the bone marrow and blood, which results in the abnormal creation of immature white blood cells. These malignant blood cells displace healthy blood cells, which causes a number of health issues. Acute lymphocytic leukemia (ALL), acute myeloid leukemia (AML), chronic lymphocytic leukemia (CLL), and chronic myeloid leukemia (CML) are the four main kinds of leukemia.

→ The effects of leukemia

Leukaemia is one of the most prevalent cancers and affects people of all ages, including both children and adults. Depending on the specific type and location, the prevalence varies.

Impact on Health: Leukaemia symptoms might range from weariness to weakness to recurrent infections to easy bruising or bleeding to swollen lymph nodes. Complications include anemia, bleeding issues, and a higher risk of infections are also possible.

Treatment Obstacles: The kind, stage, and other specific aspects of leukemia treatment vary. It frequently entails immunotherapy, targeted medicines, radiation therapy, chemotherapy, or bone marrow transplantation. The course of treatment may be lengthy and have a number of adverse consequences.

Impact on Emotion and Psychology: For patients and their families, learning they have leukemia can be emotionally taxing. Stress, anxiety, and depression might result from adjusting to treatment uncertainties, illness progression concerns, and lifestyle adjustments. Leukaemia and its therapies can have a major negative influence on a patient's quality of life. Daily activities, interpersonal interactions, and general wellbeing can all be impacted by physical symptoms, mental anguish, and treatment-related side effects.

Financial Burden: Patients and their families may have a heavy financial burden as a result of the price of leukemia treatment, which includes prescription drugs, hospital stays, and supportive care.

Research & Development: Ongoing studies and clinical trials are advancing our knowledge of leukemia and paving the way for the creation of fresh, specialized treatments. There is optimism for better treatment outcomes and an improvement in quality of life because of developments in supportive care, immunotherapy, and precision medicine.

Supportive Care: In order to improve the wellbeing of leukemia patients, supportive care and symptom control are essential. An all-encompassing approach to leukemia care must include palliative care, pain control, nutritional counseling, and emotional support.

In conclusion, since leukemia is a difficult and complicated condition that affects the bone marrow and blood, resulting in a number of health issues, self love, instead of self-pity, is the most important thing to embrace. Though it also significantly affects the family, as well as the physical and emotional health, of the patients, all hope is not lost. There are continuous studies and therapeutic developments which provide leukemia patients hope for better results and a higher quality of life. A multidisciplinary approach and supportive care are essential in meeting the many needs of patients throughout their cancer journey.

www.ingramcontent.com/pod-product-compliance
Lightning Source LLC
Chambersburg PA
CBHW071106260726
48661CB00006B/2492